VEGAN RECOVERY

By Joey Lott

www.joeylott.com

2

Publishing services provided by 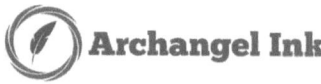 Archangel Ink

ISBN: 1518666418
ISBN-13: 978-1518666414

Table of Contents

Questioning Veganism

I know how challenging it can be to give up on veganism. I know, because I did it after being vegan for a long time. Still, I know that it was a very good choice for me. It is a choice that has offered greater health, greater peace of mind, and greater humility. My hope with this book is to offer you support in your decision to do the same.

More than two decades ago, long before veganism was part of mainstream American vocabulary, I was a 13-year-old boy in the Midwest - in the heart of meat and potatoes country - who made the switch to a vegan diet. And for 17 years, I adhered to a strict vegan diet, with the exception of a short-lived "transgression" into eating animal foods when I was 21 - something that I felt ashamed of at the time.

I believed in veganism with all my heart. I had to, in those days. I received overt hostility for my dietary and lifestyle choices from many around me at the time. I first got into veganism in the days before Google. And, in fact, I had not even heard of the Internet when I first hatched the idea. So, to say that there was little support for a lone vegan living outside of St. Louis, Missouri, in the early 1990s, would be an understatement.

My belief in veganism bordered on fanaticism, but I was quiet about my beliefs. I didn't wear 'Meat Is Murder' T-shirts. I didn't complain to non-vegans that their food disgusted me. But in my own quiet way, veganism was not unlike a religion to me. It was my moral guide. It gave me a feeling of righteousness and security. I believed that I was doing "the right thing."

But fanaticism has a way of blinding the fanatic. So it was that I didn't recognize the fallacies of veganism. I didn't realize that I was mistaken in my beliefs. I didn't realize that, in my own case, I was hurting myself in order to feel good about myself.

Finally, I made a decision that was both frightening and deeply saddening at the time. In 2010, I ceased to identify as vegan. I gave up the long-held prohibitions against eating dairy, eggs, meat, and honey. I ceased to shun leather.

In short, I dissolved the entire identity that I had clung to for all those years.

Despite the fact that it was a very difficult choice, one that I had wanted to make for nearly a year before I finally took the steps, it was a very good choice. I know it was the right choice, and I am very happy for having made it. My goal with this book is to offer you friendly support, so that you can make the right decision for you.

I am *not* saying that I know what the right decision for you is. But if you are reading this book, then I assume that you are having doubts about whether veganism is right for you, and you are reconsidering. In that case, I want to give you some information and some things to consider that may allow you to gain a wider and more balanced perspective than you have held up to now.

Let's face it: I wasn't the only one who was fanatical about veganism. And a lot of vegan literature and a lot of vegan advocates moralize veganism. So for vegans, the issue is often very heated. That makes it difficult to see the whole situation in a balanced way. Rather than trying to counterbalance the vegan bias with an anti-vegan bias, I simply want to provide a wider perspective.

I am *not* interested in converting anyone. When I gave up veganism, I gave up religion. I have no new, better religion that I want to convert you to. And I am perfectly happy for you or anyone else to be vegan, if that is your wish. I don't believe there is anything wrong with it. Even if veganism is nutritionally deficient for some people, I don't think that is a moral issue. If those people still want to be vegan all the same, then that is their business.

Despite the fact that I am not attempting to pose as a threat to vegans who wish to remain vegan, I know enough about how political veganism is to know that this book will likely receive angry reviews from those who will claim that I am a "shill for the meat industry." Which is fine. But they will be mistaken, because neither am I a "shill for the meat industry," nor am I on a crusade against veganism. I just want to offer friendly support to those who wish to give up veganism, but who are finding that they feel guilty or ashamed, or are otherwise having difficulty with the choice.

In my experience, there are essentially three main reasons that people switch to veganism and/or remain vegan: health, ethics/animal rights, and environmentalism. In what follows, we'll explore these reasons and strive to gain a broader, more balanced view of the matter in each case.

Health

Proponents of veganism for health can often cite a tremendous number of possible health benefits of a plant-based diet. In truth, most of the supposed benefits aren't specifically attributed to the vegan diet so much as they are attributed to *avoiding* animal foods. For example, many claim that animal foods cause heart disease, cancer, and other degenerative diseases. So for those who are reconsidering the vegan diet, it can be scary to contemplate eating "dangerous" animal protein, saturated fat, and cholesterol.

When I first began eating a vegan diet, I was following an extremely low-fat vegan diet because it was during the era in which the so-called health experts were claiming that fat is unhealthy. Five years later, after avoiding dietary fats as much as possible, I found myself craving fatty (vegan) foods. I remember the first time I ate an avocado. It was my first year in college. My hand hesitated as it reached for the fatty fruit in the grocery store. It felt like a violation of some sort. I didn't know if I could go through with it. But the cravings of my body won out. I purchased the avocado, and upon returning home, I halved it and plunged the spoon into the silky flesh. I ate spoonful after spoonful, until I'd eaten the whole thing.

Then I wanted more. No, I *needed* more. But I was *afraid.* I was afraid that all that fat was going to clog up my arteries and stop my heart. I was afraid I would get a stroke. I was afraid that all the terrible things that the experts had said could happen from eating fat might happen to me, if I didn't quickly curtail this transgression.

But I couldn't stop. So I ate avocadoes. Lots of them. Then nuts. Pistachios. Almonds. Cashews. For the next few years, I couldn't get enough. My poor, fat-starved body was soaking it up. But I was still afraid that by eating so much fat, I was like a ticking time bomb.

Of course, if you're not afraid of fat (and not many people are as afraid of fat these days as I was back then), then my story may seem almost comical, because fat turns out not to be so bad as we were led to believe. (Though all that polyunsaturated fat may not have been such a great idea. We'll look at that in a little while.) But what I hope to illustrate is that when we believe a story such as the "fat is bad" story, then we can be afraid of something that is perfectly fine. It was only ever just a scary story.

In the following sections, we'll explore some of the deceptions and incomplete stories that we've been told (and told ourselves) about the benefits of the vegan diet and the "dangers" of eating animal foods.

Ancestral Diets

To begin with, it is worth considering the implications of the fact that, so far as anyone knows, not a single traditional human culture has ever subsisted long-term on a vegan diet. In fact, although some groups in India and in Greece began practicing vegetarianism (though not veganism) on a larger scale, several thousand years ago, even in these cases, the percentage of the population practicing vegetarianism long-term was still fairly small.

The simple fact that, as far as we know, nearly all humans throughout history have eaten animals and animal foods should give us pause to consider why that might be so. After all, vegetarian foods are often much easier to acquire; bananas don't run away when you reach for them. So, surely, traditional people would not have worked so hard to eat animals if leaves, fruits, nuts, and tubers would have sufficed.

So what have humans traditionally eaten? Obviously, we cannot know exactly what all groups have eaten. But from the research that has been done, it appears that humans in every location have relied extensively on animal foods. And although those living closer to the equator have been able to rely more heavily on foods such as tropical fruits and coconut to provide dietary energy, the evidence is that even humans living in tropical regions have traditionally gotten substantial portions of their nutrition from fish, wild game, and livestock.

Raising animals, hunting animals, killing animals, and processing animals for food and for other purposes (such as producing leather) is not easy. It requires a *lot* of work. Not only is it physically demanding and time-consuming work, but the actual killing is not something that most people can do lightly. So why would untold numbers of humans across the globe have done all this work over all these years, if the same benefits or even greater benefits could be derived more easily through the acquisition and processing of vegan foodstuffs?

Clearly, we cannot know the definitive answer to this question. But we can assume that our ancestors had a very good reason. My guess is that they learned that the inclusion of animal foods in the diet was a necessity, in most cases. Without the animal foods, particularly in high latitudes, they found that people suffered.

Although many vegan advocates claim that there is "definitive" evidence that a plant-based diet is adequate for human health, there is simply no way to know that that is true at this point. We cannot possibly have any results from long-term studies to give us this information. What are the effects of veganism after two generations? What about 10 generations? We don't have this information. And we cannot have this information for many years, even if a study in the matter commenced today.

On the other hand, we have the implicit statements of traditional diets worldwide that say that our ancestors found the eating of animal foods to be sufficiently beneficial so as to justify the work necessary for the inclusion of these foods in the diet. And, anecdotally, we know that many cultures value animal foods for fertility and for healing.

So, although traditional diets don't *prove* that animal foods are necessary for health, neither do they offer any support to the notion that veganism is a sustainable diet for humans over time. We have at least anecdotal evidence that our ancestors have valued animal foods for health. And while they could have been wildly mistaken in their beliefs, it is notable that we do not know of a single vegan culture in all of human history.

Furthermore, all evidence is that rates of diseases that are modern epidemics, such as heart disease, diabetes, cancer, and so forth, are much lower or non-existent in most traditional cultures that have been studied. Of course, there may be other factors in traditional cultures that account for the lowered rates of disease, including more movement, less psychological stress, more fresh air, greater human community bonds, more sunlight, and so on. However, the fact that traditional diets are correlated with low rates of degenerative diseases at least suggests that animal foods, in and of themselves, do not lead unavoidably to these kinds of problems.

Cholesterol

When I was a kid, we were taught that dietary cholesterol is a killer. We were told that eggs are dangerous foods, because the yolks contain so much "dangerous" cholesterol. This view is less prominent today, but in certain circles it still has a lot of clout. So I suspect that many vegans (and non-vegans) still fear cholesterol.

Of course, while I was eating a vegan diet, I had nothing to fear when it came to dietary cholesterol, since plants don't contain the substance. But when I began to contemplate eating animal foods again, I became worried. Would all the cholesterol be harmful? Just as I had once been afraid of dietary fat, I worried that dietary cholesterol might clog up my arteries and stop my heart.

Over the years, the public conversation regarding cholesterol has become more nuanced. Whereas 20 years ago, the official line from many organizations was that all cholesterol was bad, the present conversation differentiates between so-called "bad" cholesterol and "good" cholesterol. The "bad" cholesterol is called LDL (low density lipoprotein), while the "good" cholesterol is called HDL (high density lipoprotein). And it turns out that the distinctions are even more subtle, since there are various lipoprotein particle sizes, and the particle sizes seem to produce different effects.

What is of particular note is that, in truth, neither LDL nor HDL are actually types of cholesterol. In actuality, lipoproteins such as LDL and HDL are *transporters* of cholesterol (among other fats). And it turns out that the link between cholesterol and cardiovascular disease is quite weak, because cholesterol itself does not clog arteries. In fact, what clogs arteries is something called plaque, which is produced through the oxidation of LDL and damage to the endothelium - the lining of the arteries.

The reason that LDL is susceptible to oxidation is that it is composed of polyunsaturated fatty acids such as linoleic acid, which oxidizes much more easily than saturated fatty acids. Because of this, LDL normally binds with antioxidants such as vitamin E to stabilize it. However, when these antioxidant levels are low, the LDL can become depleted and more susceptible to oxidation.

HDL, on the other hand, is said to be protective against cardiovascular disease. It is sometimes characterized as having the ability to "mop up" problems such as may be caused by oxidized LDL. And low levels of HDL correlate to high rates of cardiovascular disease.

Lipoproteins such as LDL and HDL are designed to transport cholesterol and other fats in the body. They play an essential role in health by moving cholesterol around to places in the body where it is needed. Yes, your body *needs* cholesterol.

Cholesterol is an essential component of every cell in the body, because it is used to form the cell wall. Cholesterol is necessary for the formation of myelin, which is the protective sheath around nerves.

Cholesterol is an essential component of bile, which is a substance produced in the liver that is necessary for the digestion of fats, and it is so valued by the body that it actually recycles 95% of it, rather than trying to produce a lot of new bile all the time. Plus, cholesterol is a crucial building block of essential hormones in the body – things such as progesterone, testosterone, cortisol, and so on. And finally, many researchers now believe that cholesterol plays an important antioxidant role in the body.

The cholesterol that your body needs comes either from dietary sources or is synthesized in the liver, and in other organs of the body. Your body wants cholesterol. The less dietary cholesterol you eat, the more your body will synthesize. And conversely, the more dietary cholesterol you eat, the less your body will synthesize.

So here's what we can say for certain about cholesterol. It is a necessary substance for human health. According to the current way of measuring, high levels of oxidized LDL - a damaged transporter of cholesterol - appear to be a very good predictor of cardiovascular disease.

That is about it. Despite the claims that dietary cholesterol cause cardiovascular disease, there isn't much compelling evidence that this is actually true.

There also is a growing number of researchers who now suggest that chronic inflammation may be the cause of cardiovascular disease. Of course, oxidized LDL is one possible contributor to inflammation. But so are stress, lack of sleep, extreme carbohydrate restriction, over-exercise, radiation, poor psychological adaptation, and other factors.

Another major contributor to inflammation is a type of polyunsaturated fat called omega-6 fatty acids. This is the predominant type of fatty acid found in most seed and nut oils, such as canola, corn, sesame, soy, and safflower. Although organizations such as the American Heart Association still promote the idea of substituting polyunsaturated fats for saturated fats in order to reduce cardiovascular disease risk, the evidence is mounting that most polyunsaturated fats are likely to contribute to cardiovascular disease and other types of health problems over time.

Many researchers suggest that another type of polyunsaturated fat called omega-3 has *anti-inflammatory* properties. Unfortunately, the overwhelming majority of polyunsaturated fats that many people eat, especially on the vegan diet, are high in omega-6, but low in omega-3 fatty acids. For example, almost all seed and nut oils contain very high ratios of omega-6 to omega-3, which means that the overall effect of these oils is inflammatory.

So, in conclusion, the evidence is now mounting that dietary cholesterol plays a trivial or non-existent role in cardiovascular disease. Research now suggests that the best ways to reduce the risk for cardiovascular disease include sleep, rest, reduction in stress, moderate movement (as opposed to over-exercise), and a reduction of omega-6 polyunsaturated fatty acids and oxidized fatty acids of any sort.

Saturated Fat

Saturated fat is another substance that frequently gets blamed for cardiovascular disease. Few plant foods contain large amounts of saturated fat, with the exception of tropical oils such as coconut. As such, *many* vegan diets are relatively low in saturated fat. Since many animal foods contain high ratios of saturated fat to unsaturated fat, the common advice from organizations such as the American Heart Association is to reduce saturated fat intake in order to reduce risk of cardiovascular disease. Therefore, for some who are considering eating animal foods again after having eaten a vegan diet, the fear of saturated fat may be considerable.

Let's take a look at the suggested link between saturated fat and cardiovascular disease. The American Heart Association and other organizations promote this idea because of a hypothesis put forth in the middle of the last century suggesting a causal link between saturated fat and cardiovascular disease. This link has been tenuous at best.

In studies of traditional cultures with extremely low incidences of cardiovascular disease, researchers have determined that the diets consist of large percentages of saturated fat, sometimes accounting for more than 50 percent of total calories. This fact alone casts doubt on the claim that saturated fat causes cardiovascular disease.

Many of the studies conducted over the years that are said to "prove" the hypothesis have been flawed or inconclusive. None of them were long-term, controlled, double-blind, and randomized. They often involved small sample sizes, multiple interventions, and other confounders. As far as I know, there has only been *one* long-term (eight-year) double-blind, controlled, randomized study measuring the cardiovascular outcomes when comparing diets of saturated fats versus unsaturated fats. (I am grateful to Chris Masterjohn, PhD, for his research in this matter.) That study is the Los Angeles Veterans Hospital study, which followed 846 subjects, and showed no significant difference between cardiovascular disease in the two groups.

However, importantly, the study did show a significant *increase* in non-cardiovascular deaths, mostly from cancer, in the group eating polyunsaturated fats, whereas the saturated fat group did not have this problem. Masterjohn also points out that due to the design of the study, the saturated fat group was made artificially deficient in vitamin E (most natural saturated fats are vitamin E sufficient) compared to the polyunsaturated fat group, and since vitamin E deficiency is correlated to increases in cardiovascular disease, it is possible that saturated fat was actually protective in this case. Furthermore, he also points out that the saturated fat group had a much larger number of heavy smokers than the polyunsaturated fat group, and since smoking correlates to cardiovascular disease it may be possible that saturated fat was actually protective. These last two points are speculative, but worth noting, since the evidence neatly refutes the theory that saturated fat causes cardiovascular disease.

The only other studies that I know of that are long-term and randomized (though not well-controlled or necessarily double-blind) include the Minnesota Coronary Survey (which was double-blind), Women's Health Initiative, Diet and Reinfarction trial, Oslo Heart Study, and Finnish Mental Hospital. These studies range from two years to 12 years in length, and many contain thousands of subjects. The results from each of these studies show no significant differences between consumption of saturated fat and unsaturated fat, in relation to cardiovascular disease.

Despite the claims by organizations such as the American Heart Association, there is no strong causal link between saturated fat and cardiovascular disease. And in terms of overall health, the studies are mixed. While some studies attempt to demonstrate a link between saturated fat and inflammation, others show exactly the opposite - that saturated fat may be protective against inflammation. On the other hand, there is now fairly good evidence that suggests that omega-6 polyunsaturated fats as are found in large amounts in seed and nut oils are inflammatory, which can lead to plenty of health problems.

So in conclusion, there simply doesn't seem to be any solid evidence to back up the claims that saturated fat is bad for cardiovascular health. In fact, there is better evidence that now suggests that polyunsaturated fat *may* be linked with health problems including inflammation and possibly even cancer. Those links aren't solid, either, of course. But, given the available information and the long traditions of humans eating large amounts of saturated fat, it seems to me that there is no good reason to fear saturated fat.

Can't Digest Meat

One of the persistent myths that gets perpetuated by vegan and vegetarian advocates is that humans cannot digest meat. Those who make this claim will often go so far as to suggest that meat will putrefy in the gut, creating a terribly unappetizing image. For example, PETA (People for the Ethical Treatment of Animals) makes the following claim on its website: "Meat actually begins to rot while it makes its way through human intestines." The suggestion is that this is not only unappealing, but potentially dangerous, as it gives the opportunity for "dangerous" bacteria to flourish.

But, in reality, there is absolutely no evidence to support this claim. It may have originated during times and from the same people who believed that the colon is much like a sewage system, and that it needs to be "scrubbed clean" by copious amounts of insoluble fiber and laxatives. However, the actual evidence paints a very different picture.

The stomach is a strongly acidic environment, containing hydrochloric acid as well as acidic protein-digesting and fat-digesting enzymes. The stomach environment is specific to the digestion of protein and the acidic phase of fat digestion. The acidic environment breaks down proteins into smaller parts and also acts as the first line of defense against any harmful bacteria. Then, the enzymes work to further break apart the protein into amino acids.

Meat will normally remain in the stomach for four hours, during which time it is completely broken down, in a healthy human digestive system. In fact, even large, un-chewed chunks of meat will be entirely broken down into tiny particles and amino acids in this time.

Once the stomach contents empty into the duodenum, which is the beginning of the small intestines, its pH increases so that the rest of the digestive process can occur in an alkaline environment. At this point, the bile and alkaline pancreatic enzymes mix with the contents. The bile further breaks down the fats into smaller particles and the pancreatic enzymes break down fats and any protein particles into smaller pieces - fatty acids and amino acids, respectively.

The small intestines absorb as much of the nutrition as possible during the transit time. This includes fatty acids, amino acids, sugars, vitamins, and minerals.

What passes through to the colon is only what could not be absorbed by the small intestines. In a healthy person, that will include only indigestible carbohydrates, in most cases. Unmanageable changes in diet can also produce other indigestible substances, such as fat in excess of bile or enzyme production. However, in most cases, the primary substances that pass through to the colon are indigestible carbohydrates.

By the time the digestive contents (called chyme) reach the colon, 90 percent of the water and nutrients have already been absorbed in the small intestines. The colon absorbs additional water, and whatever small amounts of vitamins and minerals may remain. The other important thing that happens in the colon is that nearly four pounds of bacteria that line the healthy human colon digest whatever they can of the remaining carbohydrates that the native human digestive system cannot digest. The bacterial digestive process produces some useful nutrients that the colon absorbs, but the majority of the bacterial digestive process feeds the bacteria and helps to form healthy stool.

Is meat rotting in the stomach or intestines at any point in this process? No, it is not. And, the only part of the digestive process that can be likened to rotting takes place when bacteria in the colon break down carbohydrates that are indigestible to humans.

So in conclusion, the "meat rots in the gut" hypothesis is nothing more than a myth oft-repeated for effect, and to push a point of view. It is has no basis in observable reality. And, in fact, meat is one of the foods that is completely digested in a healthy human digestive system.

The Digestive System of a Herbivore

Another one of the myths that gets repeated by vegan proponents is that the human digestive system resembles that of an herbivore, not an omnivore. This is meant to suggest that for humans to eat animal foods is unnatural and therefore unhealthy.

The trouble with this argument is simply that it is not true. True herbivores include cows, deer, and horses, while omnivores include pigs, chickens, and rats. So, if human digestive systems truly resemble those of herbivores, then they should be similar to cows, deer, or horses, rather than pigs, chickens and rats.

The now standard text used to support the claim that humans are natural herbivores is called *The Comparative Anatomy of Eating* by Milton Mills. This text makes many claims that range from irrelevant to utterly false.

To begin with, Mills suggests that human facial and dental structure closely resembles that of herbivores, not omnivores. However, as someone who has lived around cows and horses eating grass *all day long*, I can tell you without hesitation that humans are not even remotely equipped to chew like herbivores. After ten minutes of chewing raw vegetables, even those of us with the sturdiest of facial muscles will be aching from the over-exertion.

Next, the claim is made that only true herbivores produce saliva with the enzyme amylase, which begins the digestion of amylose, a component of starch. Since human saliva contains amylase, we are presented with the conclusion that humans must be herbivores. But this is a complete fabrication. Pigs, mice, and chickens - all omnivores - all produce salivary amylase. True carnivores, such as cats, do *not* produce salivary amylase. So the fact that humans produce salivary amylase merely points to the likelihood that we are not carnivores. But it does not rule out that we are omnivores.

Moving on, Mills claims that the pH of the human stomach is in the 4-5 range, making it only mildly acidic. He claims that omnivores and carnivores alike maintain stomach pH ranges in the range of less than 1, while he claims that all herbivores have a pH range between 4 and 5. This is misleading and false on several accounts.

To begin with, no animal maintains a constant pH in the stomach. The range will vary, depending on various factors. A full stomach tends to lower the pH because it dilutes the acids. And the amount of acid that gets produced in the stomach depends on what has been eaten. Typically, protein requires a larger amount of acid in order to digest, which can initially lower pH significantly.

Furthermore, although the ranges of pH will vary depending on various factors, the pH in the human stomach during feeding is often between 2 and 3, though it can dip down to 1 or up to 4.

Omnivores such as chickens, mice, and pigs have stomach pH ranges similar to humans, usually averaging around 2 to 3.

Cows are representative of a group of herbivores known as ruminants who have multiple stomachs, the first of which is called the rumen. In a cow, the pH of the rumen ranges from 5.7 to 7.3. Horses, on the other hand, are a type of herbivore with one stomach known as hindgut digestion. Horse stomachs have several sections that can maintain different pH values. The portion of the stomach closest to the esophagus often has a pH of 6, while the portion nearest the duodenum may have a pH as low as 2.

As you can see, the stomach pH of humans more closely resembles that of omnivores than it does herbivores.

Moving right along, Mills claims that the ratio of the length of the small intestine to the length of the trunk of the body correlates to the status of a species as carnivore, omnivore, or herbivore. He says that the ratio in carnivores is 3-6, in omnivores is 4-6, and in herbivores is 10-12 or more.

The average length of the human small intestine is 23 feet. If you assume that the length of the average human trunk is probably somewhere between 2 and 3 feet, then that would put the ratio of intestine to trunk length at around 10.

The average length of the small intestines of an adult pig will depend on the breed of pig, but an adult American Yorkshire pig (think stereotypical pink pig) has small intestines about 65 feet in length. The average length of the trunk of such a pig is less than four feet. That makes the intestine to length ratio over 15.

In rats (omnivores), the ratio is around 9. In cows (herbivores), the ratio is around 20. In horses (herbivores) the ratio is around 12. In house cats (carnivores), the ratio is between 2 and 3.

It turns out that Mills misrepresents the significance of the ratio as a correlate in this regard. True carnivores may typically have smaller ratios of intestine length to body length, and herbivores may have much larger ratios, relatively-speaking. But between omnivores and herbivores, there is considerable overlap, and this factor does not reliably predict whether a species is an herbivore or omnivore.

Finally, Mills argues that human nails and teeth make us ill-equipped to eat raw, unprocessed meat. While this argument may be compelling on the surface, it completely fails to take into account that humans make extensive use of tools for just about *everything* we do. If we were to take this argument to its logical conclusion, then we would argue that humans should not wear clothing and should not fashion shelters. More significantly, by this same line of reasoning, humans should not practice agriculture, even on a small scale. Agriculture has always required rendering land suitable for crops, the traditional approach being what is called slash-and-burn. Even this simplest form of land clearing requires the use of tools. No human can fell a mature tree without tools. Humans depend upon tools for survival whether vegan or omnivorous. Our capacity to fashion and use tools is as natural and as intimately human as our eyes, mouths, and hands.

All in all, the argument that humans are biologically and evolutionarily adapted to be true herbivores is unfounded. The evidence actually supports the claim that humans are naturally omnivores, if anything. Unlike true herbivores we are unable to extract considerable nutrition from leafy vegetables and grasses. We don't have any of the adaptations of either ruminants or hindgut herbivores. And our digestive environment is ideally suited for digesting a wide variety of foods, including animal foods.

Too Much Protein

Another persistent myth that gets frequently repeated by vegan advocates is the "too much protein" myth. The claim is that those who eat a diet that includes animal foods typically eat "too much protein," and that this results in a bunch of undesirable symptoms, including kidney damage, osteoporosis, and other baseless claims. They assert that the average Westerner eats "more than twice as much protein as is necessary," and they suggest that the vegan diet solves this problem by reducing the amount of dietary protein.

However, I have not been able to find a single study that backs up any of these claims. On the other hand, there are some studies that demonstrate that high protein diets (30% or more of calories from protein) are safe. To give you an idea of what a diet of 30% protein means, a 3,000 calorie diet would mean that you'd be eating 225 grams of protein and a 2,000 calorie diet would mean that you'd be eating 150 gram of protein. So it's a *much* larger amount of protein than what most people - meat-eaters or vegans - are typically eating on a modern Western diet.

The claim that high protein diets lead to kidney damage can be very frightening. But again, there is absolutely no evidence to support this claim, as far as I can find. On the other hand, it is not difficult to find studies (such as *Effect of a high-protein diet on kidney function in healthy adults: results from the OmniHeart trial* by Juraschek et al or *Do regular high protein diets have potential health risks on kidney function in athletes* by Poortmans et al) that measure the effects of increased protein on kidney function, and report that despite increased filtration demands on the kidneys (as would be expected), there is no conclusive evidence to suggest that protein intake leads to kidney disease. Furthermore, there is some evidence that increased protein intake does *not* lead to kidney disease (see *Dietary protein intake and renal function* by Martin et al for a good review).

What does seem to be true is that for those with existing kidney disease, high protein diets tend to exacerbate problems, while low protein diets tend to reduce symptoms. However, that does not mean that high protein diets *cause* kidney disease. To make that claim would be a bit like claiming that walking produces bone fractures in the leg because walking with bone fractures worsens the fractures. Walking with a fractured tibia may worsen the fracture, but it doesn't *cause* the fracture.

It *is* true that for *some* people with particular predispositions (which are not well-understood) whose urine has a low pH, eating large amounts of animal protein can contribute to uric acid kidney stone formation, particularly when dehydrated. Low urine pH is the strongest correlation in this case, and the solution, generally, is to maintain a urine pH that is closer to neutral rather than acidic. This is done through the inclusion of adequate fruits, vegetables, and alkaline minerals in the diet. Adequate fluids is also helpful. I add this note here simply as a caution for those who may be tempted to swing from one extreme to another by swapping a vegan diet for a low carbohydrate or ketogenic diet, which relies almost exclusively on fat and animal protein. In practice, *any* extreme diet tends to be more problematic than a moderate, balanced, inclusive diet.

The other myth that is most commonly told to scare people from eating animal protein is that a high protein diet will cause osteoporosis. The claim is that meat in particular will leach calcium out of the bones. This claim is not only baseless, but it turns out that it is the exact opposite of what a review of recent studies (*Dietary protein and skeletal health: a review of recent human research* by Kerstetter, et al) shows to be the case. The conclusion reached by the authors of the review is that "recent epidemiological, isotopic and meta-analysis studies suggest that dietary protein works synergistically with calcium to **improve** calcium retention and bone metabolism. The recommendation to intentionally restrict dietary protein to improve bone health is unwarranted, and potentially even dangerous to those individuals who consume inadequate protein."

Ultimately, though, the "too much protein" issue is a red herring simply, because an omnivorous diet does not in any way necessitate high protein intake. Let's put this in perspective. Dieticians may recommend a moderate protein diet for those who have kidney disease where "moderate protein" is defined as 1 gram per kilogram of body weight. I weigh about 180 pounds, which means that a moderate protein diet in my case would amount to 80 grams of protein per day. I happily eat liberally of both animal and plant foods, and I *rarely* eat that much protein in a day despite the fact that I eat about 3,000 calories per day.

So, in conclusion, the "too much protein" myth is just that: a myth. It is baseless and, in fact, the evidence is that there is a greater danger in eating too *little* protein versus too much. For anyone without kidney disease, it is extremely unlikely that eating animal foods will cause any problems due to a moderate increase in dietary protein.

Fiber

The conventional wisdom is that dietary fiber is good. We are told to eat more whole grains, legumes, fruits, and vegetables in order to increase our fiber intake. And we are told that refined foods such as white flour and fruit juice cause health problems specifically because of the lack of fiber.

Many vegan advocates suggest that one of the health benefits of the vegan diet is that it increases dietary fiber intake. Of course, this is not necessarily true even at face value, since it is quite plausible that one could eat a high fiber omnivorous diet or a low fiber vegan diet. But the problem with this argument goes a bit deeper. Instead of accepting it at face value, it may be beneficial to question the premise, which is that more dietary fiber is necessarily a good thing.

If we assume that dietary fiber is good and that more dietary fiber is always better, then at face value we could probably agree that a whole food vegan diet will generally provide more dietary fiber than most omnivorous diets. The trouble is that we can then make the mistake of believing that foods without fiber are unhealthy. That will necessarily lead to the conclusion that animal foods, which are almost always low in fiber, are unhealthy.

But that's a mistake. When I ate a vegan diet, I believed the "more fiber equals better health" claim, and frankly, I got lousy results after nearly two decades. But

I was so convinced of the benefits of fiber that I assumed that low fiber foods, such as animal foods, must be unhealthy. Therefore, simply because animal foods have low fiber, I was afraid to eat them.

But let's look at the reality. Is more dietary fiber a good thing? Is less a bad thing? Are low fiber foods such as meat, eggs, and dairy a bad thing?

The fiber story is much more complicated than what many of us have been led to believe. More fiber is not always a good thing. In fact, too much fiber of any kind has been shown to cause problems (for example, see *A High-Fiber Diet Does Not Protect Against Asymptomatic Diverticulosis* by Peery, et al) such as producing diverticulosis, or "pockets" in the lining of the colon. Many with various forms of inflammatory bowel disease know firsthand that some types of fiber can create further inflammation. So more fiber has a potentially dark side.

One of the major benefits that is attributed to dietary fiber is that it can help to maintain regularity. But this claim is misleading. While *moderate* amounts of *some* types of fiber have a beneficial effect on maintaining regularity, other types of fiber such as bran or rough vegetable fiber can lead to the opposite problem over time.

Soluble and insoluble fiber and other so-called "functional" fibers, such as resistant starch, pass through to the stomach and small intestine without being broken down by the innate human digestive system. Bacteria in the colon are able to eat some of these substances, though not all of them. Those that the bacteria can ferment are called, not surprisingly, fermentable carbohydrates. These feed bacteria, which can be good in balance. But like anything, too much of a good thing can cause problems. Some speculate that any excess of bulk - whether bacteria or the types of fibers that even bacteria cannot eat - can lead to problems such as diverticulosis and inflammatory bowel disease over time.

Many of us have been led to believe that insoluble fibers such as bran that resist not only human digestion but also bacterial digestion are essential to intestinal health. However, this is not necessarily true. Human feces is made up of 60-85 percent water. By dry weight it is estimated that on average (obviously this will vary greatly depending on what is eaten and other factors) about 33% is bacteria. I have yet to find a reliable breakdown by percentage of the remainder of the composition, though we do know that feces contains substances that the body secretes into the intestines in order to rid itself of them, including broken-down tissues, cells, infectious organisms, mucus, and so forth. We also know that some portion of the stool contains food that was not digested fully for some reason or another, including some types of fiber that resist digestion even by bacteria.

Indigestible fiber makes up a portion of fecal mass, but even without any indigestible fiber, humans are fully capable of producing normal, healthy stool and bowel movements. This fact, coupled with the fact that excessive fiber ingestion may cause some problems, is causing some researchers to begin to question whether more fiber is always a good thing.

When one really begins to investigate the fiber matter, it turns out that a moderate approach is probably best. There's apparently no benefit from large amounts of fiber, but moderate amounts of some types of fiber - particularly those found in fruits and some vegetables - may be beneficial. Eating a whole foods vegan diet, particularly with large amounts of bran, may be less healthful than we've been taught. But eating an omnivorous diet with a variety of fruits and vegetables is likely to provide plenty of healthy types of fiber.

I am not suggesting that the fiber issue necessarily makes an omnivorous diet better than a vegan diet. Rather, I am merely offering a different perspective on fiber that may be more balanced and more honest than what is often promoted by vegan advocates. And, because proteins and fats as are found in large amounts in animal foods are generally digested very well in the stomach and small intestine, eating these foods won't directly impact bowel health, one way or the other. However, indirectly, the fats and proteins in animal foods can provide necessary nutrition for the body, allowing for maintenance and repair of the digestive system, as well as the rest of the body.

In conclusion, eating a high fiber diet is not always a good thing. Moderate amounts of fiber or other fiber-like substances appear to be healthful, but most omnivorous diets that include even small amounts of fruit, starchy vegetables, and non-starchy vegetables will provide plentiful amounts of these healthy types of carbohydrates.

Environment

Vegan advocates now appeal strongly to our desire to "fix the environmental crisis," suggesting that eating animal foods is the cause for environmental degradation, pollution, ozone depletion, carbon dioxide levels, deforestation, and on and on. The only problem with this argument is that it is deeply distorted to push an agenda. It is not the truth.

To anyone who has ever understood rudimentary math and to anyone who has taken even a few minutes to observe the present environmental conditions in the places where we live, it is not difficult to conclude that present human civilization is not sustainable. Not only is it not sustainable, but it is railroading unbelievable numbers of other species of animals, plants, and other forms of life into terrible conditions and extinction. This much seems obvious, whether we look at the matter superficially or deeply. But the claim that the eating of animal foods is at fault for the circumstances is misleading, to say the least.

Of course, whether we can or should do something about this matter is a whole other consideration. But for the purposes of this book, I am going to assume that you believe that it is preferable to improve conditions and change the apparently destructive habits of human civilization. In that context, it is sensible to ask two questions. First, is veganism an effective way to achieve that goal? And secondly, is an omnivorous diet inherently opposed to that goal?

In what follows, I would like to take a look at some of the common arguments that are made as to why veganism is an environmentally-friendly way of life, and why the eating of animal foods is a threat to environmental integrity and health. For each of these arguments, we will then examine them and try to see if we can answer these questions about the pros and cons of veganism and omnivorism.

Greenhouse Gas Emission

In 2006, the United Nations released a report that vegan advocates like to point to as damning evidence against animal foods. The report puts forward the suggestion that livestock worldwide account for a staggering 18% of greenhouse gas emissions *measured in CO_2 equivalent*. On the surface, this would suggest that eliminating livestock in the world would immediately reduce 18% of greenhouse gas emissions. But this is misleading. And, furthermore, it is a red herring, as we will see shortly.

To begin with, how is it that the UN special report could diverge from the numbers of other reports worldwide, such as the U.S. Environmental Protection Agency's report that claims that 10 percent of (U.S.) greenhouse emissions are from all of agriculture, including both livestock and the cultivation of plant foods? It turns out that it does not. In fact, the UN numbers are essentially the same as those from the EPA, but the UN report plays with the numbers. The key phrase in the report is "measured in CO_2 equivalent." What that means is that, in the UN report, the 18 percent figure weights the methane production of livestock 23 times more heavily than carbon dioxide output since, in a certain light, methane can be considered to be 23 times more powerful as a greenhouse gas when compared to carbon dioxide.

While I don't wish to offer a complete critique of the UN report, the 18 percent figure is highly suspect to me on account of, by most estimates, livestock account for about 9 percent of methane production while the rest is produced primarily by other human activities such as industry, landfills, and mining.

But just for the sake of argument, let's run with the 18 percent figure. So we will assume that worldwide livestock account for 18 percent of the effects of greenhouse gasses. Okay. Fine. But to jump from that to the conclusion that eating animal foods is harmful to the planet or that veganism is more environmentally friendly is too big a leap. Let's break it down a little bit.

To begin with, it is essential to consider that these numbers are for *conventional livestock production*. The UN report details at length the implications of fertilizer use for grain and soy production, diesel-powered farm equipment, stored manure, and other factors that apply *only* to animals raised in confinement and fed unnatural diets of grain and soy.

Now, I've seen plenty of feedlots. I've *smelled* feedlots. I've seen the runoff. I've seen cows packed into small spaces, heads between bars, chowing down on grain in a trough. It's not a pretty picture - or smell. But it is disingenuous to suggest that confinement animal feeding operations (CAFOs) are the only way to produce animal food, or that alternatives would have the same environmental effects.

I live among many small homesteads and small farms that raise 100 percent grass-fed sheep, goats, or cows, and the result is night and day different than CAFOs.

Grass-fed herbivores require absolutely no input of grain or soy. Their manure is used as fertilizer and is not even mildly offensive. And these small operations do not necessarily require any fossil-fueled farm equipment.

Humans have been keeping livestock for thousands of years. Some estimate that cows may have been domesticated as far back as 30,000 years. And during the overwhelming majority of the time that humans have kept livestock, they required no vast input of fossil fuels, no feedlots, and no erosion or runoff. In fact, many now argue that reverting natural grassland back to prairie and grazing livestock on it may actually *improve* the environmental situation.

So superficially, if we were to assume that all livestock has to be raised on grain and soy in CAFOs, then it would be *less* environmentally damaging for all humans to stop eating animal foods and to instead eat more plant foods. That would theoretically allow for less land to be used not only for livestock, but also for agriculture in general. So it's a nice theory on the surface, but if we are instead comparing grass-fed animals, then it's a very different story. And there are compelling arguments suggesting that it may be more environmentally friendly to eat locally-raised, grass-fed animals than to eat large amounts of agricultural products that may have been transported great distances.

Fundamentally, the argument for veganism because of the possible flaws of *any* method of raising livestock is totally off the mark. That is because livestock is not the only viable source of animal food available to humans. Wild animals are not only a plausible source of animal food, but for the overwhelming majority of human history they have been the *only* source. And to omit wild animals from the discussion is a major oversight.

Wild animals such as deer, moose, bear, rabbit, beaver, raccoon, and so on require absolutely no input from humans or human systems. They do not depend on agriculture. And they require no deforestation. And because they eat their native diets when living in wild places, they are likely to provide optimal nutrition as food, as compared to CAFO-raised animals.

Finally, the argument that veganism is an effective way to improve environmental conditions is disingenuous. Even if we accept the 18 percent figure offered by the UN report, that leaves 82 percent still to look at. So how do we account for the other 82 percent of human-related greenhouse gas emissions and effects? Well, according to the EPA's numbers (which figure that agriculture as a whole accounts for 10 percent of emissions), industry accounts for 20 percent, electricity for 32 percent, transportation for 28 percent, and commercial and residential for 10 percent. If we really want to go after the worst offenders, then the most genuine environmentalist would not waste time with livestock. Instead, she or he would demand the immediate cessation of all electricity generation, all industrial production, all industrially-powered transportation (cars, trains, planes, etc.), and all other fossil fuel use such as natural gas or propane use. And, as it turns out, in tackling those issues, we would also necessarily dramatically reduce the greenhouse emissions from livestock since, naturally, there would be no more large-scale agriculture, chemical fertilizer use, or any feasible way of managing a CAFO.

The UN report masquerades as an indictment of livestock, but it fails to point the finger at the real culprits: industry, industrial agriculture practices, and greed.

In conclusion, the indictment of animal foods on the grounds of the UN report is misguided. Industrial agriculture and industrial livestock practices are both unethical and unsustainable. But it is disingenuous to claim that eating animal foods is inherently environmentally damaging or that veganism is a solution to the perceived problem.

Water

The UN makes the claim that 13,000 to 15,000 liters of water is required to produce a single kilogram of cow. This is compared to 1,000 to 2,000 liters required to produce a kilogram of wheat. Vegan advocates like to hold these sorts of facts up as damning evidence against the eating of animal foods. Of course, if humans were capable of living off of wheat alone and if the 13,000 to 15,000 liter per kilogram of cow figure were accurate, then it *would* be rather damning. So let's investigate and see what is really going on.

The actual UN report makes an important qualification of the statement that is often omitted in discussions among vegan advocates. That key qualification is that the numbers apply to the production of *grain-fed* beef. So how is this number calculated? Well, the 13,000 to 15,000 liter per kilogram figure is based upon the amount of water necessary to produce the amount of grain that is necessary to feed a cow in order to produce a kilogram of live cow. Sources vary in terms of how much grain (in kilograms) is required to produce a kilogram of beef, but on the high end, we get a figure around 8. (Note that the numbers increase to around 20, if we are looking at weight of muscle meat alone.)

So, it is not difficult to see how taking these numbers together, we can arrive at a figure such as 13,000-15,000 liters of water. However, this number is *only* applicable for grain-fed CAFO cows. If we look at grass-fed cows grazed on natural pasture, then this requires zero grain input. The only water input for grass production is rainfall.

Already we can see that the water argument used against the eating of animal foods is *really* an indictment of industrial agricultural practices, not animal foods. Natural, grass-fed livestock raised on small homesteads or small farms do not require obscene amounts of water to produce food.

But there's much more to the story. For one thing, despite the criticisms of the water usage for (grain-fed, CAFO) animal food production, other reports from the UN indicate that other commonly-used *vegan* products require *significantly* more water. For example, by weight, roast coffee requires nearly 33 percent more water than beef to produce and a cotton t-shirt requires nearly twice as much water to produce as the equivalent weight in beef. Plus, according to the UN report, even milk from grain-fed cows requires *far* less water to produce than wheat, soy, or rice. Eggs require less water to produce than rice. So the vegan advocates are cherry-picking from the reports to support their cause, which is disingenuous.

What is more, in addition to sustainably-raised livestock, there are other environmentally-friendly options for eating animal foods, which include wild game. As I have pointed out before, wild animals require no industrial input of any kind nor do they require any deforestation. They are the ultimately environmentally-friendly food, which is a fact that vegan advocates and a great many environmentalists neatly leave out of the discussion.

But there's still more. According to U.S. Geological Survey estimates, in the United States, the two largest uses of water are thermoelectric power (49 percent of total) and agricultural irrigation (31 percent). Next comes public supply (11 percent). The remainder of water usage is tiny in comparison. And the amount of water that is used *directly* for livestock? Less than one percent.

So the true environmentalist who is concerned with water usage would be far more concerned with water used by thermoelectric power generation and agricultural irrigation than the water used for livestock. Granted, some percentage of the water used to irrigate agricultural fields indirectly is being utilized by CAFOs, but truly, it is the industrial agricultural practices that should be falling under scrutiny, not the eating of animal foods.

In conclusion, the argument that livestock water demands is a valid reason to reject animal foods is unfounded. Grass-fed livestock produced locally and wild game are environmentally-friendly animal food sources. The true culprit revealed by the reports is not animal food, but industrial practices across the board.

Pollution

By now, most of us have heard of the horrors of agricultural pollution, such as the annual "dead zones" in the Gulf of Mexico that blot out most life forms in the region. Vegan advocates like to blame these atrocities on meat consumption, but the arguments are weak.

The claim is that waterways are being polluted directly by runoff from CAFOs, such as manure and unmetabolized antibiotics and growth hormones that are routinely fed to confinement animals. Furthermore, some blame animal food for pollution from tanneries and chemical fertilizers and pesticides used to produce grain to feed CAFO animals.

But these criticisms have nothing to do with animal food. They have everything to do with industrial practices.

One of the major complaints is that animal manure runoff in waterways accounts for massive amounts of excess nitrogen. This excess nitrogen is harmful to native species in the water, but it feeds algae, which are perceived to be problematic in a variety of ways. But this argument falls flat on its face when we consider that one of the major chemical inputs in agriculture is nitrogen! In the case of chemical fertilizers, the nitrogen comes from petroleum, but farmers for thousands of years have known about and relied upon nitrogen and other benefits of manure, also sometimes called "black gold." So the problem here is not manure itself, nor the raising of animals for food. Instead, the problem is unsustainable industrial practices and the mismanagement of an otherwise valuable product - manure.

The arguments against raising animals for food because of the introduction of unmetabolized antibiotics and other drugs into the environment is likewise an indictment of industrial practices, rather than raising animals for food. Humans have raised animals for thousands upon thousands of years without any need for antibiotic drugs or growth hormones. The introduction of these chemicals into livestock production coincides with CAFO popularity. But still, small farms and homesteads have no need to rely on these drugs. Naturally raised livestock is still a very viable (and sustainable) option.

Likewise, as we've already seen, grass-fed animals require no agricultural input, which renders moot the argument against animals as food because of the unsustainable practices of industrial agriculture.

Plus, once again, livestock is not the only viable option for animal food. Wild game is, as always, a perfectly environmentally-friendly food source.

In conclusion, the rejection of animal foods on the grounds of pollution is misguided. In fact, the blame for pollution can be more honestly pinned on industrial practices of all kinds. Meanwhile, naturally-raised, grass-fed livestock and wild game are environmentally-friendly food sources.

Erosion and Habitat Destruction

Finally, yet another common argument used to blame meat consumption for environmental problems is that modern livestock production causes soil erosion, deforestation, and habitat destruction.

Once again, this argument is not really a fair critique of animal foods. Rather, it is an argument against industrial practices and irresponsible choices. While it may be true that CAFOs produce soil erosion, the *opposite* is often true of small-scale raising of grass-fed livestock. In many cases grass-fed cattle are known to *improve* the quality of land and reduce erosion significantly. Some even argue that converting Midwestern corn fields to pasture for cattle would be a dramatic environmental improvement by reducing erosion and actually sequestering carbon.

There is a dark side, even to grass-fed livestock, unfortunately. The Brazilian government estimates that 80 percent of the Amazonian deforestation is the result of clearing of land to make pasture for grass-fed cattle. And this goes to show that, like anything, too much of a good thing isn't so good. So while modest, local grass-fed livestock production is likely sustainable, greedy, environmentally-damaging practices such as clear-cutting rainforests for pasture is a terrible idea.

Still, the environmentally-damaging practices of some does not mean that eating meat is inherently environmentally unfriendly. As it turns out, the native humans who have lived for thousands of years in the Amazonian rainforest that is now being clear-cut have eaten omnivorous diets, subsisting in large part from animal foods. And, as far as we can tell, their practices were not damaging to the environment.

Wild game remains, as always, a viable food source, and one that requires no deforestation.

In conclusion, raising livestock responsibly does not cause erosion. In fact, it may reduce erosion and help to sequester carbon. While modest, local, sustainable livestock production is environmentally-friendly, it is also important to keep in mind that it is not the only source of animal foods. Wild game remains the most environmentally-friendly of all.

Meat in the Environmental Debate

Finally, let's wrap up the discussion of the environmental impacts of eating meat and other animal products. The bottom line is that we have pretty good evidence that humans have lived for hundreds of thousands of years while relying on animals for food. And during the vast majority of that time, it would seem that they did so in a sustainable fashion. It is only since the advent of agriculture that we have evidence that human activities have made significantly negative impacts on environmental health, and the impacts seem to have increased dramatically with the advent of industrial activity.

When we look at the bigger picture, it seems that eating animals is not incompatible with environmental health. Rather, it would seem that human overpopulation, large-scale agricultural practices, and industrial activities are the problems.

In the discussion, vegan advocates often like to argue that the amount of grain used to produce CAFO beef could instead feed hundreds or even thousands of humans. This argument is, sadly, an anthropocentric view that places humans as the highest priority.

If we truly look at the bigger picture, and if our primary concern is for the well-being of not only humans but non-human animals and other life forms, then the argument that veganism can help to feed more humans turns out to be not so compelling. The evidence is pretty strong now that human populations have grossly overshot the natural carrying-capacity of the planet. What that means is that feeding more humans with vegan diets may prolong the inevitable reduction in human population, but it may come at a terrible cost - the mass extinction of even more species.

In other words, if we are to define veganism as a compassionate outlook that considers the health, well-being, and intrinsic rights of all beings, not just humans, then feeding more humans with a plant-based diet is actually incompatible with the essence of veganism.

It seems to me that a true environmentalist will look at the bigger picture and see where the greatest leverage can be found. Converting the world to a plant-based diet is unlikely to offer great leverage. Instead, a look at the numbers indicates that the biggest offenders are electricity production, cars, planes, trains, buses, and industrial agriculture. Given that, the true environmentalist would be taking action to bring about the end of these practices.

It is tempting, of course, to want to seek out a sense of personal environmental purity - to feel that you are "doing your part" by eschewing meat, using less water at home, and riding your bicycle more often. But while these things may offer a feeling of righteousness, that's about all they provide.

I understand that the environmental argument in favor of veganism is one that can be difficult to let go. It requires humility - the recognition that the answers aren't always so simple as making the "right" choices in our personal lives. And that includes what we eat personally. The fact of the matter is that the public debate has been skewed in favor of industry and the maintenance of industrial lifestyles, such as living with electricity and cars. But in truth, when you look at the big picture, what we each eat individually is insignificant and is largely a product of the context in which we live. If we are truly concerned about making a difference, then we would be best off making changes in the greater context, rather than worrying about the trivialities of what we ate for lunch or whether we wear leather shoes.

Ethics

The ethical argument in favor of veganism is, perhaps, on its surface the most compelling argument made for giving up meat, dairy, eggs, honey, leather, and so on. Most of us desire to be kind, to be loving, to treat all forms of life with respect. Many of us have looked another species in the eye and seen that there is life there, not so different from human life. We form relationships with dogs, cats, rabbits, horses, cows, and all types of other species. And we love them and wish them a good life.

The problem with the ethical argument in favor of veganism is just that it is superficial. It completely ignores or overlooks the complexities of life and death. So in the following sections of the book, I'd like to scratch beneath the surface and examine the interconnectedness of life and death, and the insincerity of the "meat is murder" argument.

Food Cycle

All of life is interconnected. None of us are separate. In fact, what we call our "environment" becomes indistinguishable from ourselves when we look closely enough. With each breath, we are changing inside for outside and outside for inside. Moisture escapes from our skin. Food and drink become flesh and bone, and flesh and bone become urine and feces. The distinction between inside and outside is difficult to keep track of, especially the closer one looks.

Despite the fact that modern practices distort our view of things, the reality is that humans are intimately connected with everything. For example, for hundreds of thousands of years most humans saw directly how their urine and feces that fell to the ground were eaten by bacteria, fungi, plants, and animals, providing nourishment that keeps the cycle going. In truth, there is no such thing as waste because the output from one organism is the input for another. Each of us helps make nutrients available for other species.

In the vegan ideal, none of us would ever do harm to another. And, superficially, this is a noble cause. But when we begin to see the interconnectedness of all of life, this ideal gets fuzzy. In what way can I truly ensure that I am doing no harm? By what standard do I measure harm? Am I taking into account the bigger picture?

If I truly wish to do no harm, then I must honor the natural cycles. There are beings who are depending on me to feed them. My sweat, blood, and tears, as well as my urine and feces, are needed by other beings. If I withhold them, then that is a form of harm. Likewise, someday my body will begin to decompose rapidly and it will then be food for billions upon billions of other species ... if they are allowed access and the body is not tucked away inside a sterile box.

Whether I eat fungus, bacteria, plant, or animal, I am ingesting a form of life. This is how I participate in the natural cycle. All food is life. It is life changing form and continuing the cycle.

So then the question is, how can I best honor the cycles? How can I best feed those who count on me? How can I best support those who feed me? And keep in mind that I am fed not only by the foods that I eat, but by the air I breathe, the water I drink, and all sensory inputs, including sights and sounds. We humans need more than just calories, vitamins, and minerals. We need wild places and wild beings to sustain us.

My own answer to these questions is that it is not so simple as "eat a plant-based diet." In fact, when considering the bigger picture, I'm not convinced that a plant-based diet is best. For reasons that we've seen earlier in the book, and for reasons that we've yet to explore, I suspect that a vegan diet may require more habitat destruction, more species depletion, and more pollution than an omnivorous diet that makes use of sustainably-raised livestock and wild game, along with sustainably-raised plant foods and wild plant foods.

Is eating an animal inherently wrong? Is it wrong to kill another for my sustenance? If we are locked into a false paradigm that views life and death as polarized opposites, then these questions can be neatly answered – yes, it is wrong to kill. But life and death aren't actually polar opposites. They are connected through a cycle. Death marks a transition from one form to another, but it is one life.

When I eat, whether I eat a carrot or a cow, that form changes. But it is a continuation of the cycle of life. My body, as I conceive of it, is constantly in flux. As much as 90 percent of the cells in my body are bacteria - not strictly human. And those cells are changing often as many billions of bacteria exit the body every time I defecate. Along with the billions of bacteria cells, each poop also includes cells that were formerly muscles or organs or blood. Lymph and mucus also exits with each excrement.

All of that goes on to feed bacteria, fungi, plants, and animals who feed upon what I excrete. This is particularly evident if I am more closely connected with land, adding my humanure and urine to the soil. The nutrients that I give to the land feed the land, which feeds others. Those others feed still others. And on and on until I am fed once again, keeping the cycle going.

Hairs fall from my body. Skin cells shed. This too feeds the land or, in the case of hair, may be used temporarily as bedding or nesting material by others, giving comfort to those who are also part of the cycle just like me.

In the bigger picture, we are all part of the cycle. Our importance or value is not greater or lesser simply because of our size or our mobility, or our taxonomy.

From the larger perspective, a human is no more important than a lettuce plant, and a cow is no more important than a wasp. We are all one in the cycle. Can we honor that? Can we trust that?

Unfortunately, the vegan story is often founded upon the assumption of human supremacy. But, if we drop the notion that humans are superior to, say, dandelions or oak trees, then perhaps a new perspective can emerge. Is the killing and eating of animals actually wrong? Or, is it possible that when we step back and take our place in the cycle, that moderate, sustainable, and respectful killing and eating of animals is natural and balanced?

If we truly wish to restore balance and ethical treatment of all of life, might we not see other paths that may give us more positive leverage, in that respect, than blindly eschewing animal foods in order to take the moral high ground? Perhaps, instead of striving to end all killing of animals, we might endeavor to end the production of electricity, the use of industrially-powered modes of transportation, and industrial practices of all kinds. We might seek to restore land to the wild. And we might seek to take our place in the cycle of life, rather than trying to step outside of it.

Indirect Slaughter

For ethical vegans, the very idea of slaughter can make one a bit queasy. But it is a mistake to take the moral high ground and believe that a vegan diet absolves one of complicity in mass slaughter.

In 2008, I had been vegan for about 16 years, and one day, out of the blue, it suddenly occurred to me that the carrot that I held in my hand came at a cost of many lives. I realized that the cultivation - even small-scale organic cultivation - of carrots or other vegan foodstuffs required the death and displacement of untold numbers of living beings, small and large. For a field to exist requires that the life forms that would otherwise exist there - trees, ferns, grasses, deer, elk, salamanders, frogs, etc. - have to be killed or displaced.

The land is alive, and that life is intimately connected. There exist trillions of tiny organisms within a small sample of soil. There are complex mycelial networks that span vast distances, connecting the plants and animals throughout the region. The plants rely upon the mycelia and the bacteria for their survival, sometimes even depending on them for uptake of nutrients. The plants feed and often house insects and other types of organisms. The animals are mobile, carrying food, insects, seeds, nutrients, and information of all sorts over relatively long distances. All are interconnected.

All of that is disturbed to grow food. To grow a carrot requires many deaths and much destruction. The field has to be maintained and cultivated each season. So the disturbance is ongoing; the deaths are ongoing.

Estimates suggest that as many as 75% of the animals living in a field - of which there are many, including mice and rabbits among others - are killed during harvesting in large-scale industrial operations. And even on a small scale, the animals may be killed.

Pesticides range from chemicals used in industrial farming operations to natural products used by small-scale organic gardeners to human hands killing insects. I've worked on organic farms and grown food myself, and I can tell you that oftentimes the choice is between killing large numbers of animals (often insects) or losing the crop. As an example, in New England, potatoes are often infested with thousands of beetles and their larvae. If allowed, they will completely devour the plants, leaving nothing to produce the edible tubers. The solution? I've been recruited by organic farmers to pull Japanese potato beetles off the plants, one at a time, place them in jars, and then close the lid on a jar of hundreds of insects, allowing the heat of the sun to cook them to death because the chickens don't even want to eat them.

The point here is that, even on the small scale, production of vegan foods means that many others have to be killed in order to keep the crop. There is no escaping it.

Of course, if we each grew all of our own food, then we could still not escape the necessary displacement of other beings nor the necessary killing of others in order to save the crops. But we could at least eliminate the costs associated with food transportation. However, for most of us, simply eating a vegan diet doesn't eliminate this aspect of how food gets to us.

Vegan food from all over the world is transported by truck, train, plane, or boat, making its way to our grocery stores, natural food stores, and food co-ops. Even if we purchase food at a local farmer's market, the food still travels to the market by truck. And the simple fact is that these modes of transportation necessitate the slaughter of vast numbers of beings. Produce is shipped to New England from California by trucks that therefore must drive thousands of miles on highways, killing untold deer, raccoons, opossums, foxes, dogs, cats, mice, birds, and what must amount to a gazillion insects.

The simple fact is that a vegan diet is likely to necessitate the indirect slaughter of so many animals that the difference between a vegan diet and an omnivorous diet in this regard may be insignificant.

Of course, I am not suggesting that CAFOs are ethically sound, because by most any standards they are not. But once again, the point I want to make is that it is a mistake to conflate animal foods with CAFOs, because they are not synonymous. Ethically-raised animals and wild game offer a viable, ethical source of food

And finally, if our true concern is the ethical treatment of animals of all kinds, including fish, insects, birds, reptiles, amphibians, and mammals alike, then eschewing meat is too simplistic. It is a complex matter. We could take it to the extreme like the Jain monks who sweep the path before them to brush aside insects so that they are not stepped on. But we could also discover a more mature approach and acknowledge that every action that we take, even the simple action of breathing, involves the death of countless beings. Death is part of the cycle of life.

Then, instead of just trying to take the moral high ground, we can begin to investigate how it is that we can live in such a way as to truly honor all of life by honoring death. Then, each breath may become an act of gratitude for those who are meeting death in this simple, natural, and unavoidable act. Similarly, the act of eating can become an act of gratitude and thanksgiving, honoring and acknowledging that whether we are eating potato or beef, many have met death in order that we might be nourished by this meal.

Parting Words

Veganism is a noble idea in many regards. But that doesn't make it correct. The trouble we can get ourselves into is believing that veganism is the one true way that will save our health, save the environment, and give us the moral high ground. This can lead to unpleasant righteousness, judgment, frustration, zealotry, and so on. And furthermore, if and when you begin to have doubts about whether the vegan way is the right way for you, you may experience guilt and shame for not being able or willing to make veganism work.

My hope in this book is that I have given you a broader perspective and invited you to question the stories that claim vegan superiority. Whatever you choose in your life - vegan or not - I hope that you can do so with peace and humility, knowing that your choice is simply that: a choice, and not a moral imperative.

If you have found this book to be liberating, please do not make the mistake of turning this into a new form of zealotry - anti-vegan zealotry - because that is not my intention. Even though I am convinced that the vegan claims are mistaken, I don't believe that there is any type of moral imperative to *give up* veganism! I simply see it as a choice that is free of morality.

Upon reading this book, if you find support for a choice to eat an omnivorous diet, then I encourage you to get to know your food. Even though I raise and produce a relatively small amount of my food, I have found that the experience of raising, slaughtering, and processing some of my own food has given me a deep connection with all of my food. It has offered me a new-found respect for all that I eat.

And finally, whatever you take from this book, if nothing else, please accept the invitation to be gentler with yourself and with others. Instead of feeling that the burdens of the world are placed squarely on your shoulders, I invite you to relax and find the joy of humility, acknowledging that none of us has a monopoly on truth. It is noble to desire to "do the right thing" - to be conscious, loving, and caring. It is a beautiful thing to wish to end suffering and help to create and maintain balance in the world. But perhaps this book has helped you to discover that our ideas of what all of that should look like aren't always right. Truth, to whatever degree there is such a thing, is far beyond the capacity of the human identity to capture. The rules that we create are not absolute truths. And personal purity and perfection, though it may create a feeling of righteousness, isn't necessarily beneficial in a broader sense.

The intricacies and balances of life are vast and well beyond our individual capacities to control or understand. May we all discover true peace. May we all discover balance. May we all love so deeply that we are willing to take our place in the cycle of life and death.

Get My Future Books FREE

If you enjoyed this book (Hey, if you made it this far it couldn't have been that bad), you'll probably enjoy many of my other books about health and wellness. And you can get all my new releases in health and wellness for free by signing up for my mailing list at www.joeylotthealth.com. It's simple, it's free, and it's totally honest and legitimate. Nothing scammy or spammy or anything else like that (i.e. I won't be trying to sell you The 7 Dirty Underground Top Secret Weird Tricks for Rock Hard Abs or Young Living Oils). It's just about free books for those who appreciate my work, because I appreciate YOU. Simple as that.

Connect with Me

I welcome your questions, comments, and feedback of any kind. Please feel free to email me at joeylott@gmail.com. I am now receiving so many emails that I cannot always reply to every email. I do read them all, and I do my best to reply to as many as possible. For the benefit of others, I may choose to publish my response to your email on my blog or in book format. I will maintain your privacy and anonymity if I choose to publish my response.

One Small Favor

My sincere goal in writing is to share something that may be of value to you. And I endeavor to do so while keeping the costs low for readers. The success of my books and my ability to reach other readers who may benefit from my books depends in large part on having lots of thoughtful, honest reviews written about my work. You would do me a great favor if you would please take a moment to generously write a review of this book at Amazon.com. This will only take a few minutes of your time, and you will be helping me a great deal. I sure would appreciate it.

Free Video Series

I also have a site at www.peacefulpossibility.com where I have over three hours of free video training on a handful of limbic system retraining techniques, including the Big Chill. On that site I share more detailed instruction. Everything on the site is completely free. Nothing is for sale there.

About the Author

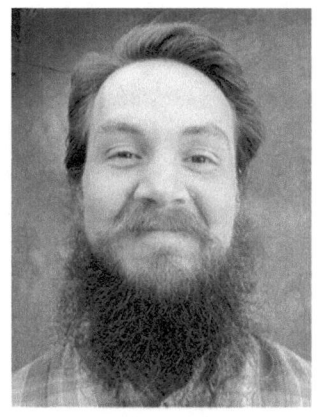

"The secret to happiness is to let go of everything - see through every assumption."

Beginning at a young age Joey Lott experienced intensifying anxiety. For several decades he lived with restrictive eating disorders, obsessions, compulsions, and an inescapable fear. By the time he was 30 years old he was physically sick, emotionally volatile, and mentally obsessed with keeping any and all unwanted thoughts and experiences at bay.

At this time Lott was living on a futon mattress in a tiny cabin in the woods. He was so sick that he could barely move. He was deeply depressed and hopeless. All this despite doing all the "right" things such as years of meditation, yoga, various "perfect" diets, clean air, and pure water.

Just when things were at their most dire, a crack appeared in the conceptual world that had formerly been mistaken for reality. By peering into this crack and underneath all the assumptions that had been unquestioned up to that moment, Lott began a great undoing. The revelation of this undoing is that reality is utterly simple, ever-present, seamless, and indivisible.

Lott's books provide a glimpse into the seamless, simple, and joyous nature of reality, offering a glimpse through the crack in conceptual worlds. Whether writing about the ultimate non-dual nature of reality, eating disorders, stress, disease, or any other subject, he offers the invitation to look at things differently, leaving behind the old, out-grown, painful limitations we have used to bind ourselves in suffering. And then, he welcomes you home to the effortless simplicity of yourself as you are.

Not sure where to begin? Pick up a copy of Lott's most popular book, *You're Trying Too Hard*, which strips away all the concepts that keep us searching for a greater, more spiritual, more peaceful life or self.